The Little Library of Healing Herbs

Astrologicals

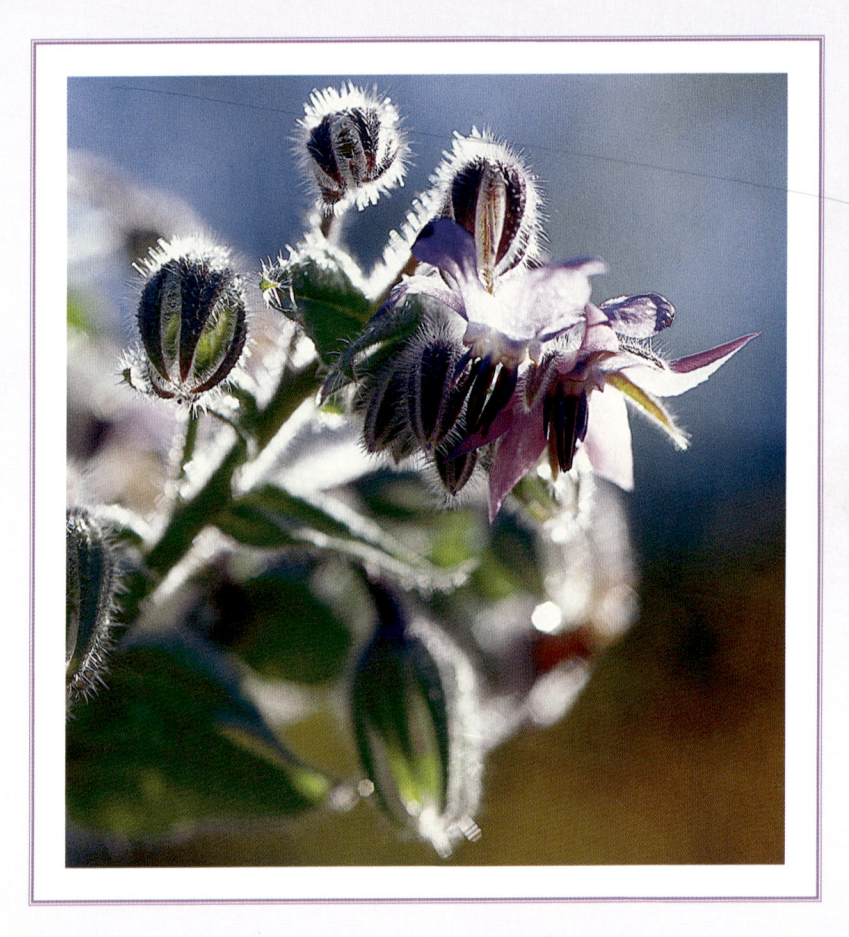

The Little Library of Healing Herbs

Astrologicals

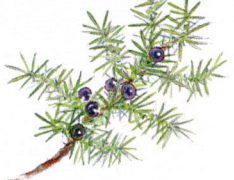

PAST TIMES

PAST TIMES

www.past-times.com

This edition published by PAST TIMES in 2004

01 03 05 04 02
1 3 5 7 9 10 8 6 4 2

The Little Library of Healing Herbs was created and produced by
Carroll & Brown Publishers Limited
20 Lonsdale Road London NW6 6RD

Written and compiled by Ian Wood
with thanks to Joanna Watters
Copyright © Carroll & Brown Limited 2004

A CIP catalogue record for this book is available from the British Library

ISBN 1-903258-97-9

All rights reserved. No part of this publication may be reproduced in any material form (including photocopying or storing it in any medium by electronic means and whether or not transiently or incidentally to some other use of this publication) without the written permission of the copyright owner, except in accordance with the provisions of the Copyright, Designs and Patents Act of 1988 or under the terms of a licence issued by the Copyright Licensing Agency, 90 Tottenham Court Road, London W1P 9HE. Applications for the copyright owner's written permission to reproduce any part of this publication should be addressed to the publisher.

Reproduced by RDC, Malaysia

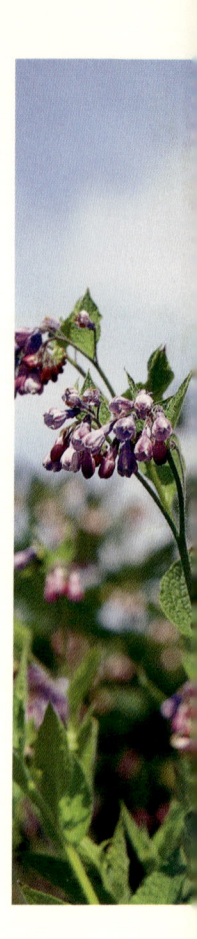

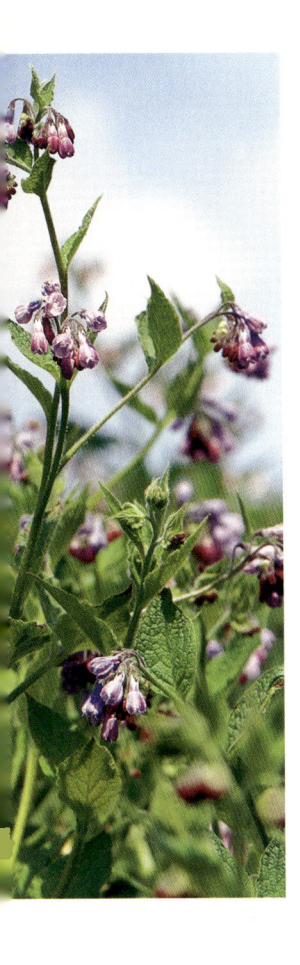

Contents

Introduction 6
Culpeper's Herbal 8
The Sun – Leo 10
Juniper 12
The Moon – Cancer 16
Mercury – Gemini and Virgo 20
Peppermint 22
Venus – Taurus and Libra 26
Mars – Aries and Scorpio 32
Jupiter – Pisces and Sagittarius 36
Dandelion 38
Saturn – Capricorn and Aquarius 42
Sunflower 46
Making Infusions and Decoctions 48
Herb Glossary 54
Herbs in Your Garden 58
Growing Herbs Indoors 60
Harvesting Herbs 62
Index 64

Introduction

Herb Safety

Please note that although herbs are natural products and most are safe to use, in some circumstances they can have harmful effects. If you have any allergies or other medical conditions, if you are pregnant or breastfeeding, or if you are taking any form of medication (including oral contraceptives), consult your doctor or a herbalist before using any herbal remedy.

People have known about the healing properties of herbs for many thousands of years, although until the rise of modern science they had no way of knowing exactly how or why they work. But early herbalists did have an explanation for the effectiveness of herbal medicine, which fitted the facts as they saw them, and their theory was based on astrology.

According to this theory, the Sun, the Moon, and the planets each ruled specific organs of the body. They also ruled the herbs that had proved to be effective remedies for the ailments of those organs. Jupiter, for example, ruled the liver, so if someone had a liver complaint, a herbalist would prescribe one of the herbs of Jupiter (such as dandelion) to cure it. So this theory provided an explanation of how herbal medicine worked, and a useful way of classifying medicinal herbs and their uses.

7 ASTROLOGICALS

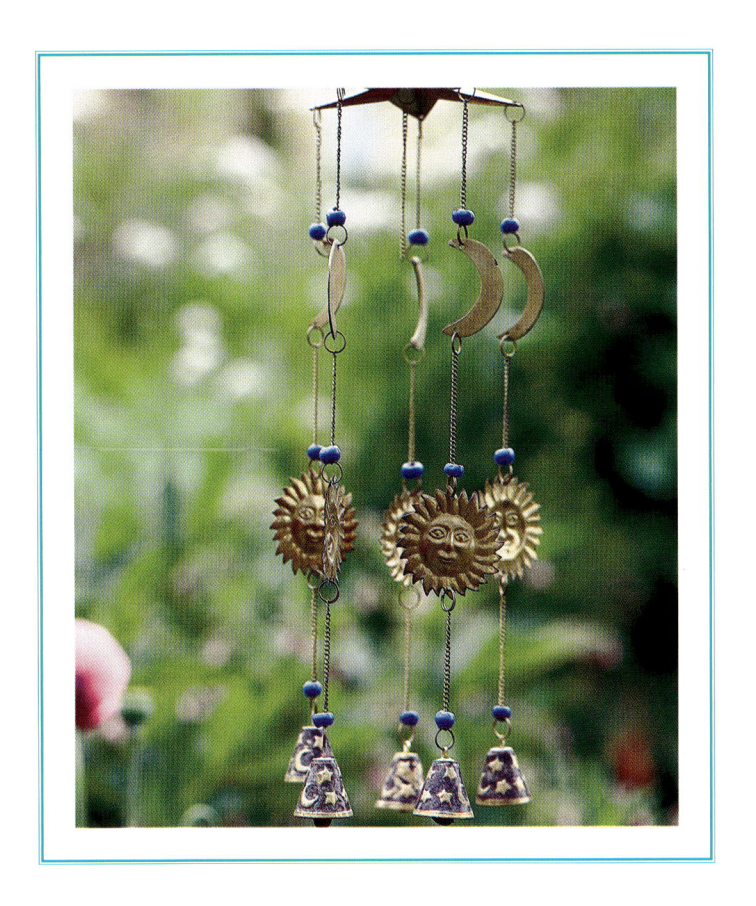

Culpeper's Herbal

MUCH OF WHAT WE KNOW about the ancient link between astrology and herbal medicine is based on the work of an English herbalist called Nicholas Culpeper (1616–1654). By Culpeper's time, the medical profession was beginning to discard the astrological background to the theories of medicine and herbalism, and he believed that this was a great mistake.

After two other influential herbalists of the time, John Gerard (1545–1612) and John Parkinson (1567–1650), published works on herbalism that ignored the astrological theories, Culpeper produced a book that he hoped would reverse this trend. This book, which is now his best-known work, was *The English Physician Enlarged*, or *The Herbal*. Published in 1653, it included information about how the planets influence both our health and the curative properties of herbs, and became an instant best-seller that helped to preserve ancient knowledge that otherwise might have been lost to us.

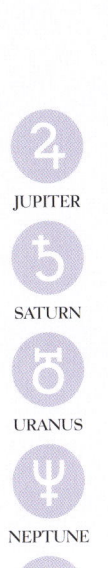

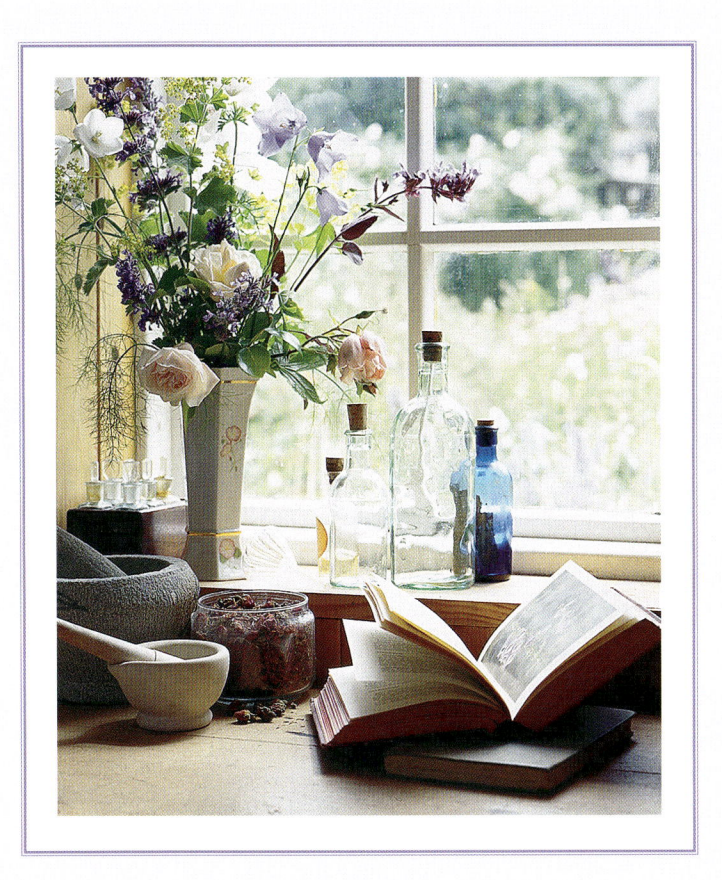

♃ JUPITER	♎ LIBRA
♄ SATURN	♏ SCORPIO
♅ URANUS	♐ SAGITTARIUS
♆ NEPTUNE	♑ CAPRICORN
♇ PLUTO	♒ AQUARIUS
	♓ PISCES

9 ASTROLOGICALS

The Sun – LEO

LEGEND & LORE

In traditional Icelandic folklore, it was believed that juniper and rowan trees could not grow close together because each created so much heat that they would destroy each other. For the same reason, it was thought that bringing juniper and rowan sprigs together into a house would cause it to burn down.

IN TRADITIONAL ASTROLOGY, the Sun is known as Lord of the Day and it symbolizes vitality, consciousness, and the ego – how we embrace life and experience our sense of self. The Sun rules the right eye in a man and the left eye in a woman, and both the Sun and Leo (July 23–August 21) rule the heart and the back, in particular the spine, so Leos tend either to have excellent posture or back problems.

The Sun and Leo also symbolize royalty, stateliness, warmth, and passion. Their colours are gold, yellow, and orange and the Sun's metal is gold, and some of the solar plants – for example sunflower, saffron, orange, lemon, heart trefoil, and marigold (*calendula*) – directly reflect this symbolism in their names. Because the Sun is essential to life, the herbs of the Sun, such as juniper, are considered to be sun-seeking and life-giving.

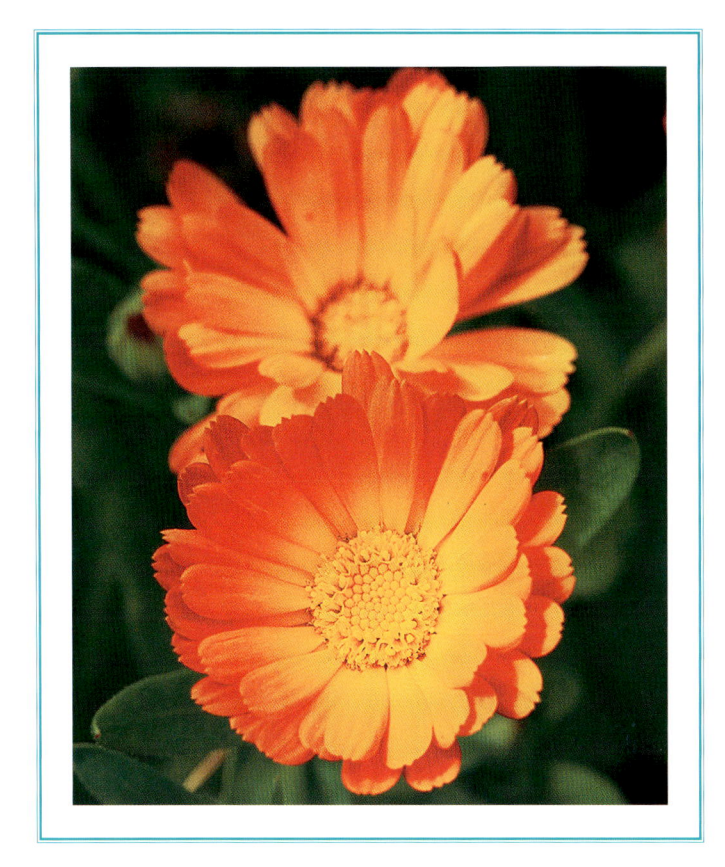

Calendula

Juniperus communis

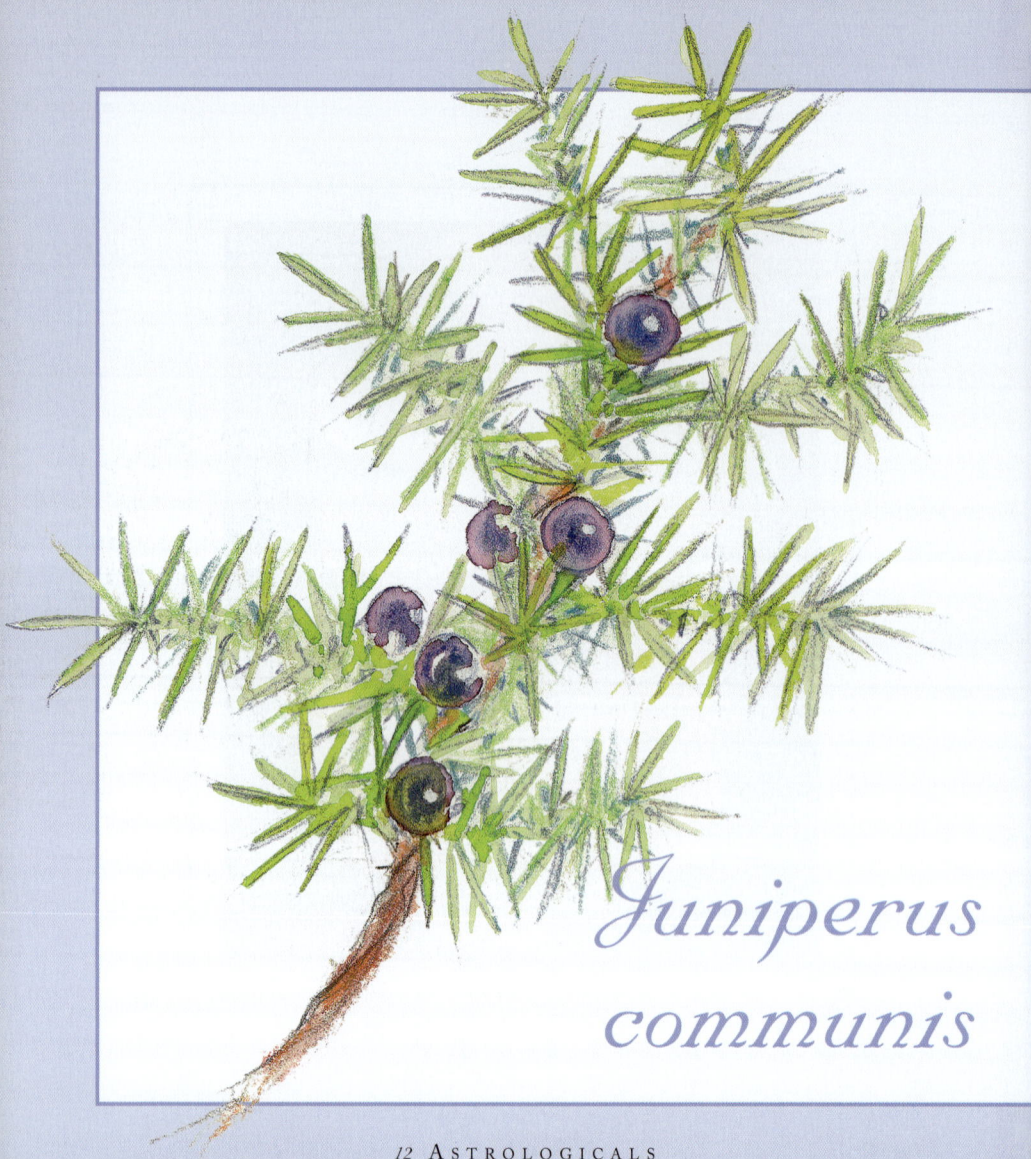

Juniper

*J*uniper is an evergreen shrub, widely distributed throughout the Northern Hemisphere. In Norse mythology it was sacred to Thor, the god of thunder and the sky, and the Celts used to burn juniper wood or berries to purify the air and drive away evil spirits.

The shrub has needle-like leaves and usually grows to a height of about 180 cm/6 feet, and its berries change colour from green to blue or purple as they ripen, a process that takes two or three years. Ripe berries are harvested in September and October for use in herbal medicines and to flavour foods and drinks. The berries are used in herbal medicine for urinary tract disorders, rheumatism, neuralgia, and joint and tendon problems, and in cooking they are used as a seasoning in sauerkraut and for adding a spicy flavour to meats, especially venison. Juniper berries are also the principal flavouring ingredient of gin.

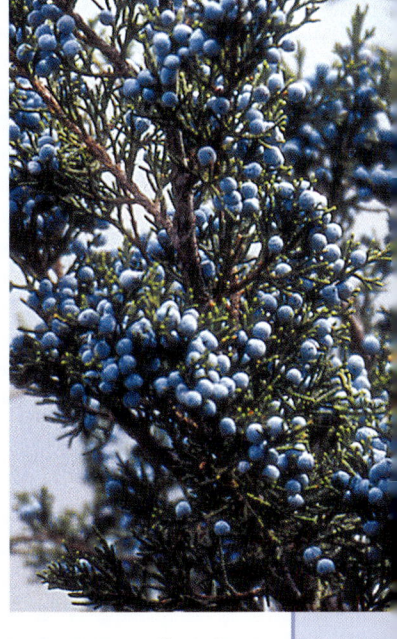

14 ASTROLOGICALS

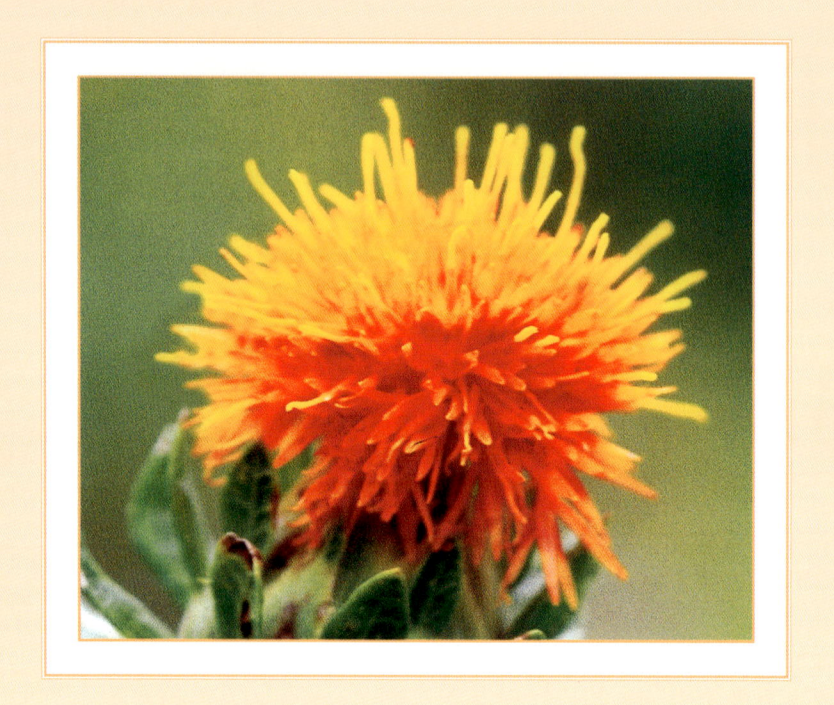

> "Let the hot sun
> Shine on, shine on."

W H Auden
Let the Florid Music Praise
1936

The Moon – CANCER

TRADITIONALLY THOUGHT OF AS FEMININE and known as the Lady of the Night, the moon holds sway over all that is unconscious, habitual, or shadowy, and represents our feelings, needs, and emotional responses. Her twenty-eight day cycle reflects the menstrual cycle, and she rules over womanhood, pregnancy, fertility, babies, and motherhood. She also rules the breasts, the right eye in a woman and the left eye in a man, and because she is the ruler of the stomach, people born under her sign of Cancer (June 22–July 22) may be prone to nausea and stomach upsets.

Both the Moon and Cancer symbolize a nature that is protective, nurturing, receptive, and retentive, and their colours are silver and white. Lunar herbs include those considered to be cooling, drying, or sleep inducing, and herbs such as coriander (*Coriandrum sativum*) and ginger that act as tonics for the stomach.

> **THE HERBAL CABINET**
>
> Ginger originated in Asia, and is widely grown there, but most of the ginger sold around the world today comes from Jamaica. The plant was brought there by the Spanish in the sixteenth century, and grown on plantations for export back to Europe.

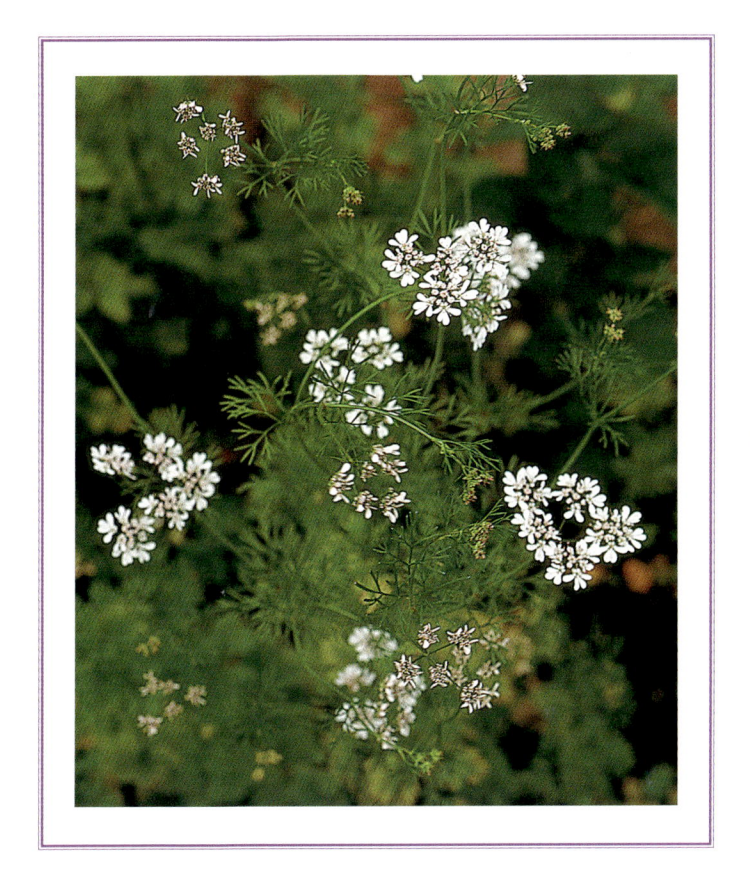

Coriandrum sativum

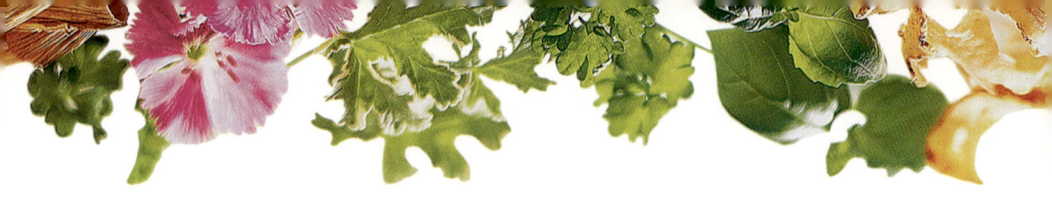

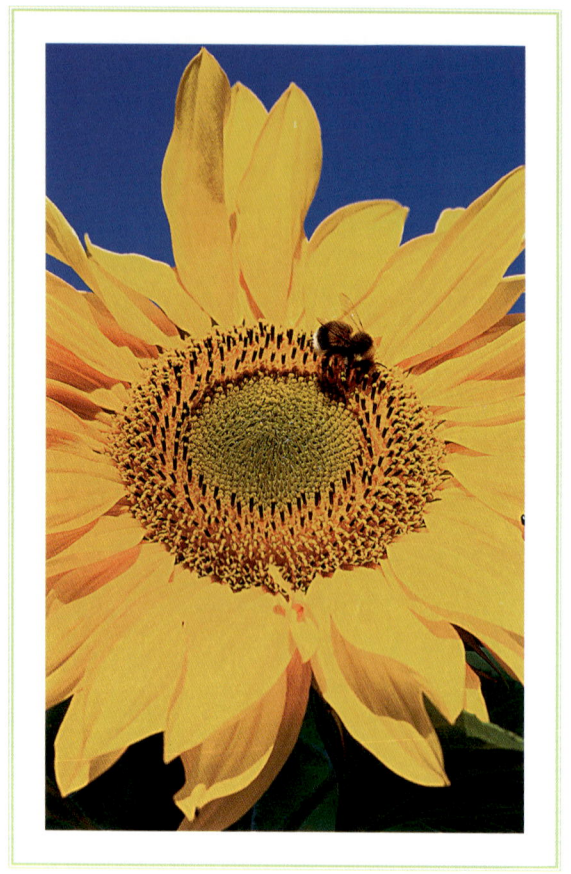

18 ASTROLOGICALS

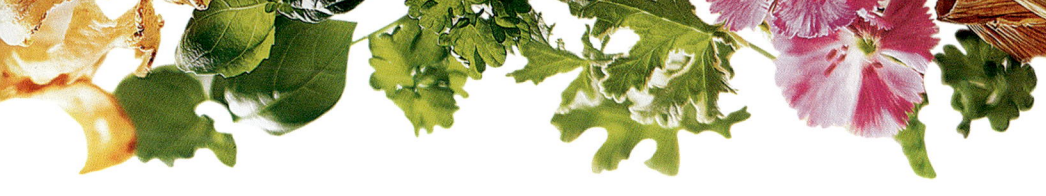

Juniper and Sunflower Massage Oil

120g/4oz crushed juniper berries
1 litre/2 pints sunflower oil

To soothe an aching back or tired muscles, massage the affected area with an infused oil made with fresh juniper berries. Add the crushed berries to the sunflower oil. Pour the mixture into clear glass containers, leave them in a sunny spot for 15 days, then strain and use.

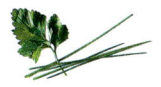

Comfrey Poultice

A comfrey poultice can help heal broken bones, sprains, and minor flesh wounds, and ease the pain of arthritis.

large handful fresh comfrey leaves
boiling water
flour

Crush the fresh comfrey leaves, add just enough boiling water to cover them, and leave them to soak until soft. Mix the flour and more water into a paste, add the comfrey leaves, combine thoroughly and apply the paste to the affected area while it is still hot, using a clean cotton cloth or bandage to hold it in place. Leave it there until the poultice has cooled.

Mercury – GEMINI and VIRGO

THE PLANET OF THE MIND, Mercury rules everything to do with thought, communication, and expression. Its masculine sign, Gemini (May 22–June 21), rules the nervous system and the shoulders, arms, and hands, so Geminis tend to be changeable, restless people who often gesticulate energetically as they talk. It is easy to see why people born under this sign are prone to anxiety and nervous exhaustion, and why Mercury's herbs include the mildly sedative valerian (*Valeriana*).

> **THE HERBAL CABINET**
> Valerian, an important ingredient of many herbal sedative preparations, has an odour that most people find unpleasant but is powerfully attractive to many animals. Cats, for example, love to roll around on valerian plants, and rat-catchers used to bait their traps with it.

Mercury's feminine sign, Virgo (August 22–September 23), is the perfectionist, embodying the mind's rational functions of discriminating, analyzing, and defining. Virgos tend to have a strong work ethic but they are also the zodiac's expert worriers, and, as this sign rules the intestines, the stresses felt by Virgos are likely to bring on digestive problems. Peppermint, made into a tea or an infusion, is a pleasant and effective remedy for indigestion.

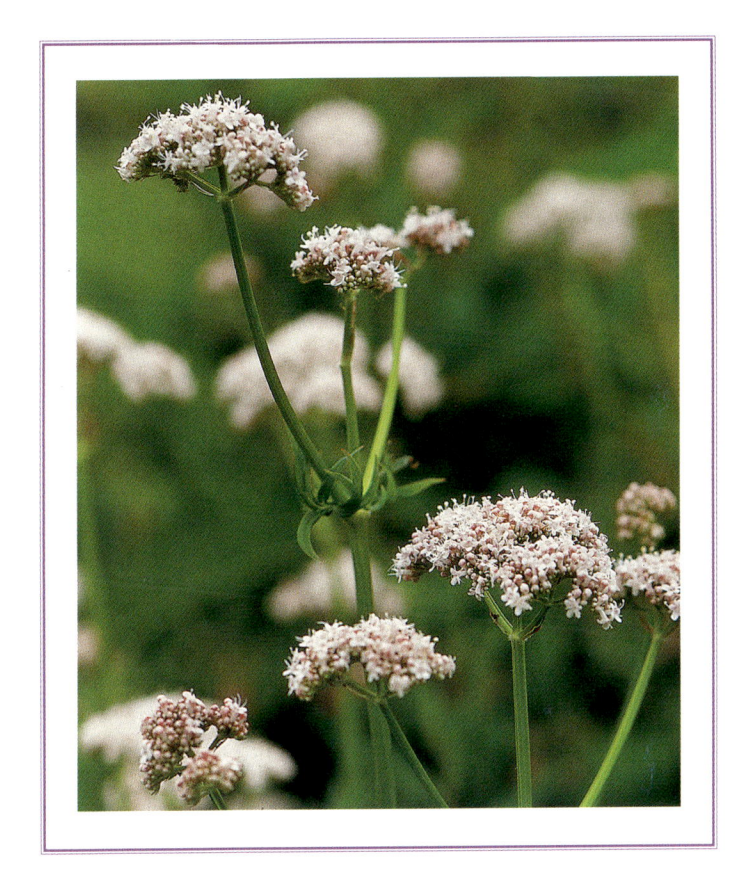

Valeriana

21 ASTROLOGICALS

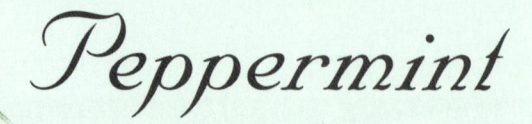

Peppermint

Peppermint is a hybrid of water mint (*Mentha aquatica*) and spearmint (*Mentha x spicata*), and its use as a medicinal and culinary herb dates back 3,000 years or more to the days of the ancient Egyptians. It was also popular with the Greeks and Romans, and according to a Greek legend the first mint was created after Pluto, god of the underworld, fell in love with a nymph called Minthe. His disgruntled wife, Persephone, changed Minthe into a plant, and although Pluto could not undo the spell, he was able to give the plant its well-known and distinctive sweet scent.

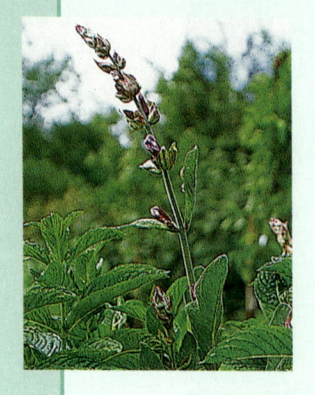

Peppermint is a spreading plant that grows 30 to 60 cm/1 to 2 feet high, but can reach 90 cm/3 feet when in bloom. Its leaves contain a volatile oil rich in menthol, which is peppermint's main active ingredient and is mainly responsible for the herb's flavour and its soothing and antibacterial properties.

Mentha x piperita

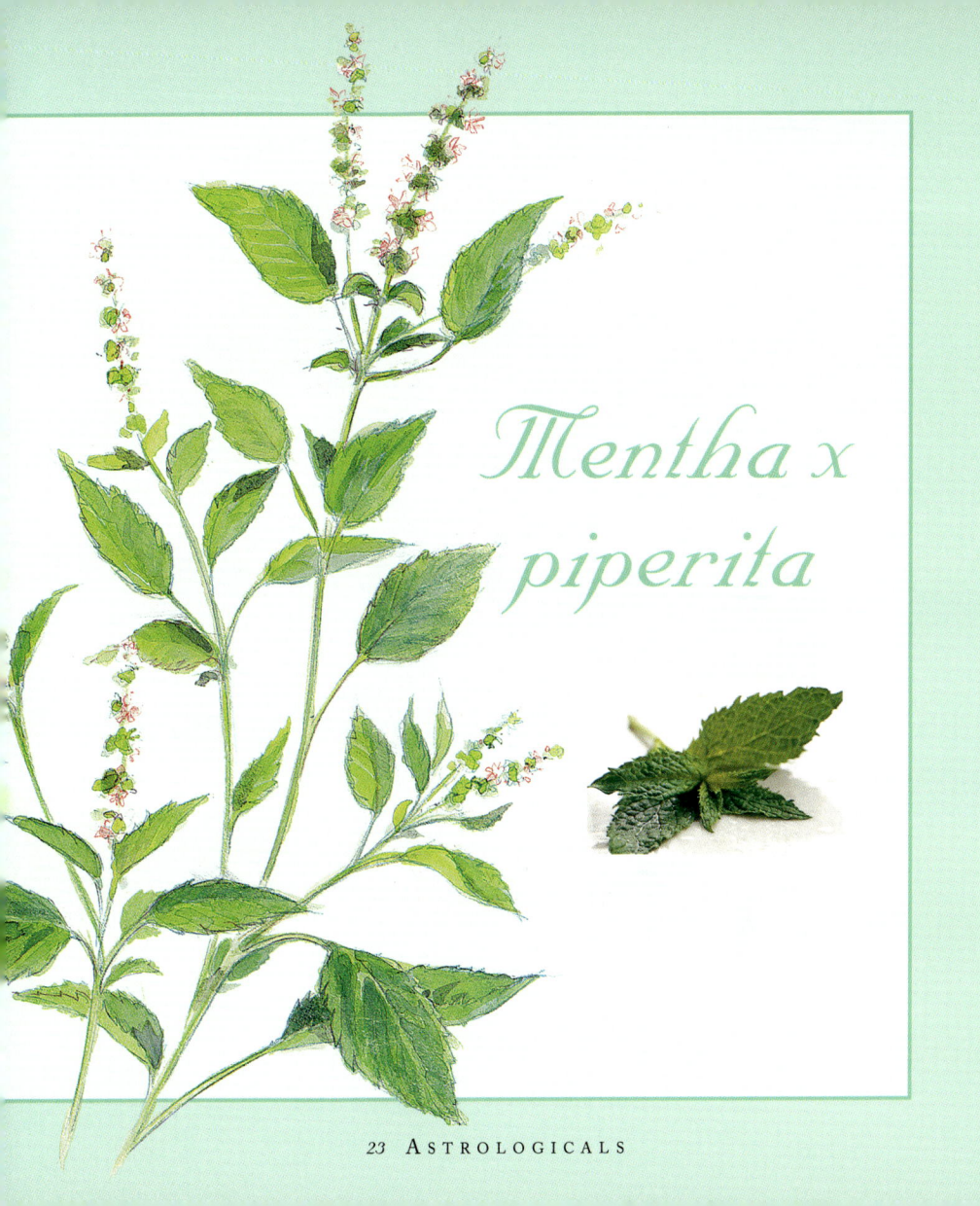

23 ASTROLOGICALS

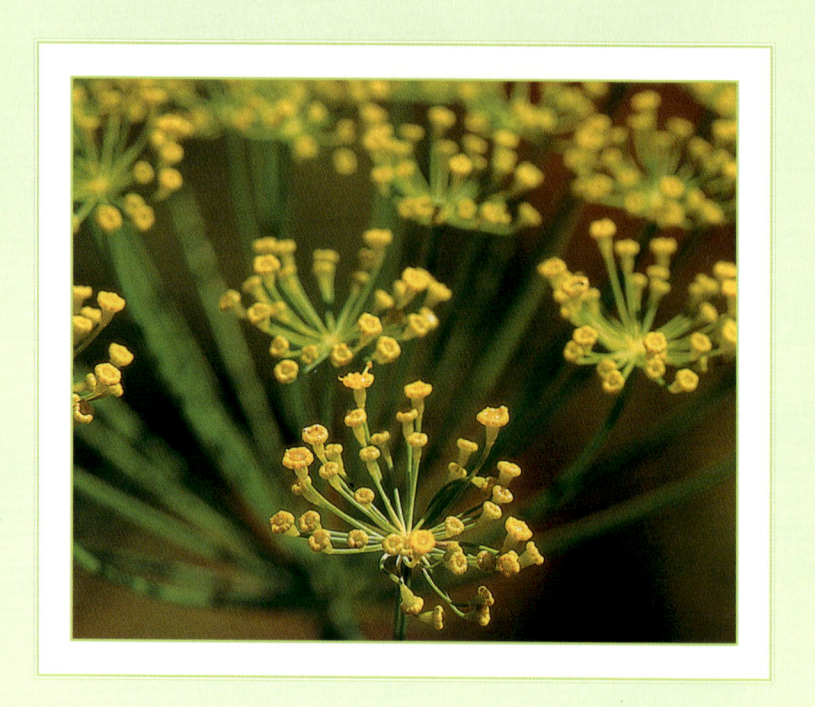

"My father named me Autolycus; who being, as I am, littered under Mercury, was likewise a snapper-up of unconsidered trifles."

WILLIAM SHAKESPEARE
THE WINTER'S TALE
1610–11

Venus – TAURUS and LIBRA

IN TRADITIONAL ASTROLOGY VENUS is the planet of love, romance, marriage, and partnership, and Venusian herbs include sweet, fragrant flowers such as roses, along with more robust plants such as mallows and burdock. Venus' feminine sign is earthy Taurus (April 21–May 21), which in turn is the sign of food, money, materialism, and possessions. The way to a Taurean's heart is without question through the stomach, but in physical terms Taurus actually rules the neck and throat. This sign is especially vulnerable to sore throats, which can be soothed by an infusion of marshmallow leaves.

> **THE HERBAL CABINET**
>
> Burdock is so named because its leaves are like those of the dock plant and it produces burrs, seed cases covered in tiny, hook-like hairs. These burrs latch onto anything that rubs up against them, and in 1948 Swiss inventor George de Mestral (1907–1990) came up with the idea for Velcro after picking burdock burrs off the fur of his dog.

Venus' masculine sign is Libra (September 24–October 23), which in turn is the sign of partnership, balance, and diplomacy. Libra rules the kidneys and Librans are especially prone to kidney infections, so regular detoxing with a small glass of fresh burdock (*Arctium lappa*) leaf juice can be particularly beneficial for this sign.

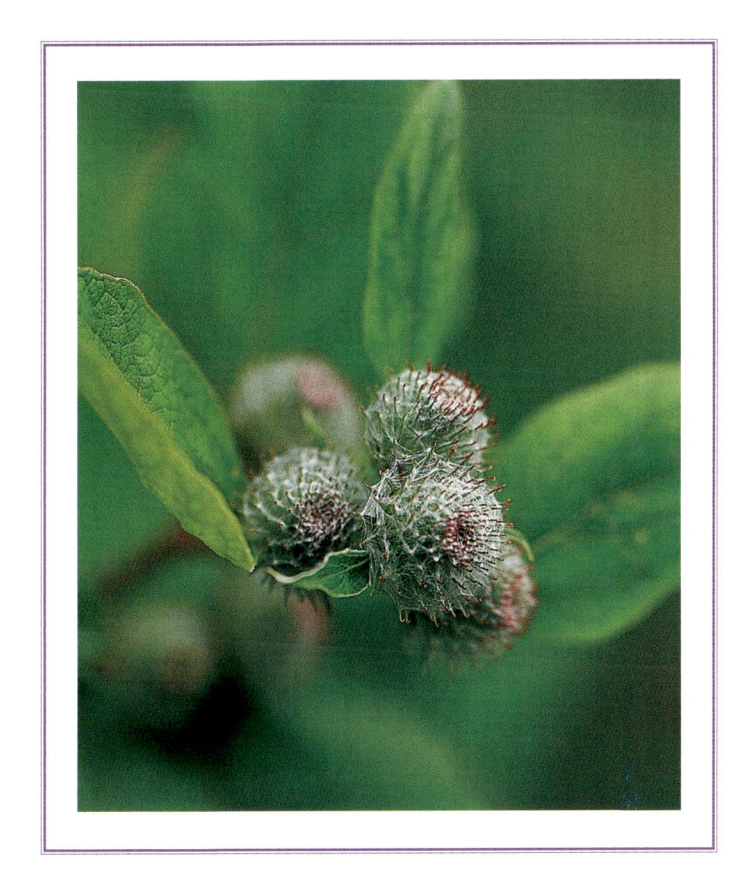

Arctium lappa

27 ASTROLOGICALS

28 ASTROLOGICALS

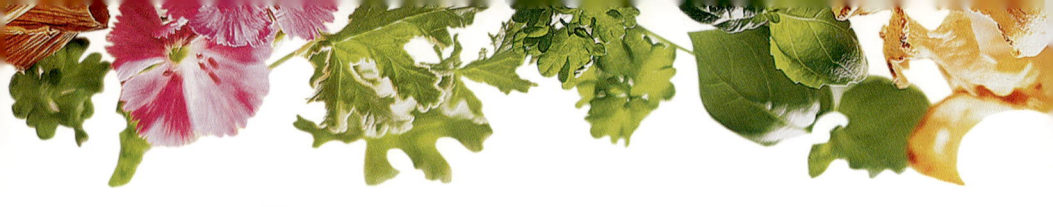

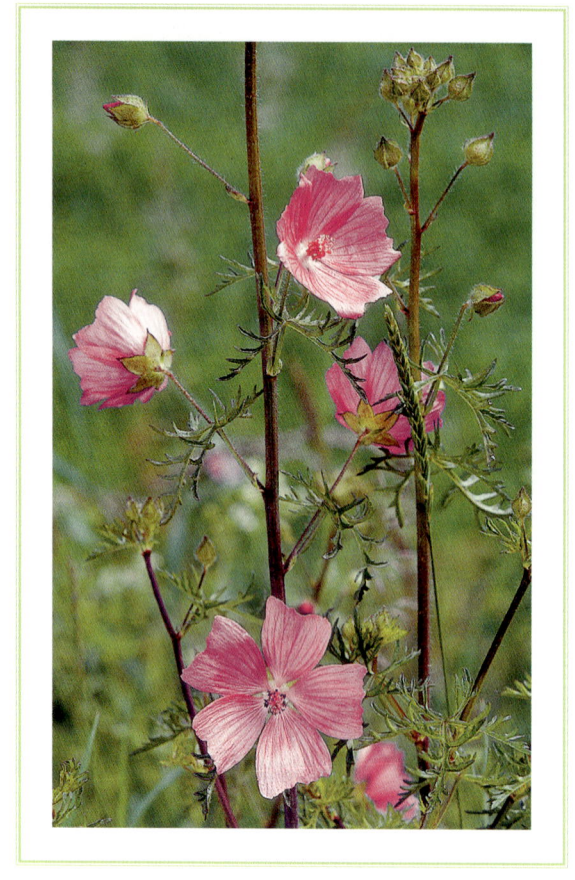

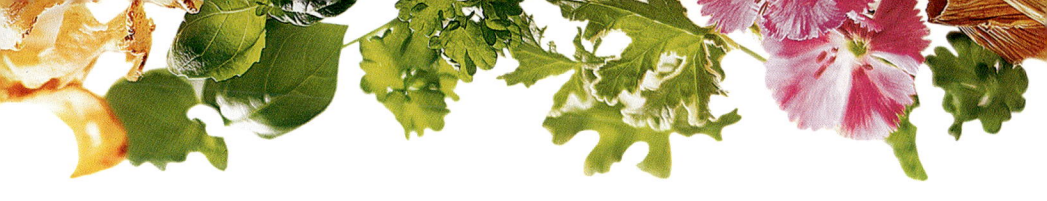

Marshmallow Gargle

A cold infusion of marshmallow provides effective relief for a sore throat.

4 tbsp fresh marshmallow leaves
600 ml/1 pt cold water

Put the fresh marshmallow leaves into the cold water and leave to steep for 8–12 hours. Strain out the leaves and use the liquid as a gargle three or four times a day.

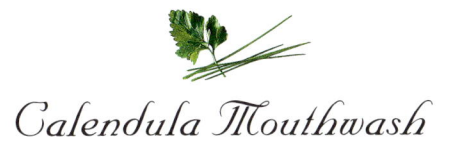

Calendula Mouthwash

Calendula is antiseptic and astringent, and is especially helpful for treating mouth ulcers and gum disease.

1 to 2 tsps dried calendula
boiling water

Simply add the dried herb to a cup of boiling water and allow to steep for 10 minutes. Strain out the leaves and use this as a mouthwash three or four times a day.

30 ASTROLOGICALS

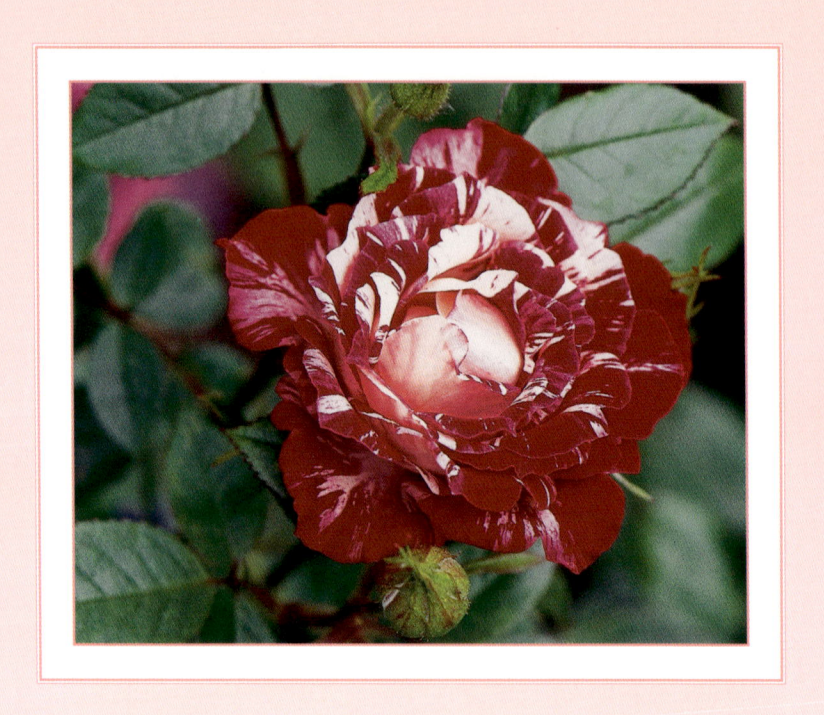

"To Paris the other goddesses might have seemed lovely,
But, compared with those beside her, Venus won.
Don't just compare the face, but their characters and skills:
So long as love doesn't cloud your judgement."

OVID
REMEDIA AMORIS
C. 5 BC

Mars – ARIES and SCORPIO

LEGEND & LORE

The ancient Greeks believed that rocket was a very effective aphrodisiac, and they used to plant it around their statues of Priapus, god of fertility. The Romans also believed in rocket's stimulating qualities, and in many parts of the Roman Empire people ate it in salads to counteract what they believed to be the passion-killing effects of lettuce.

IN MYTHOLOGY MARS is the god of war, so the planet Mars symbolizes men, battles, weapons, energy, courage, anger, and aggression. These qualities are embodied in Mars' masculine sign of Aries (March 21–April 20), the warrior of the zodiac, and the Aries personality is quick, direct, and impatient. At the physical level Aries rules the head and face, so afflictions including headaches, migraines, and sinusitis can be treated with herbs that belong to Mars, such as plantain (*Plantago*).

Scorpio (October 24–November 22), Mars' feminine sign, is known for its famous sting in the tail and love of power. Mars symbolism is reflected in Scorpios' incomparable determination and their ability to cut to the heart of the matter. Scorpio rules the reproductive system and sexual organs, and rocket, another of Mars' herbs, is said to have aphrodisiac properties.

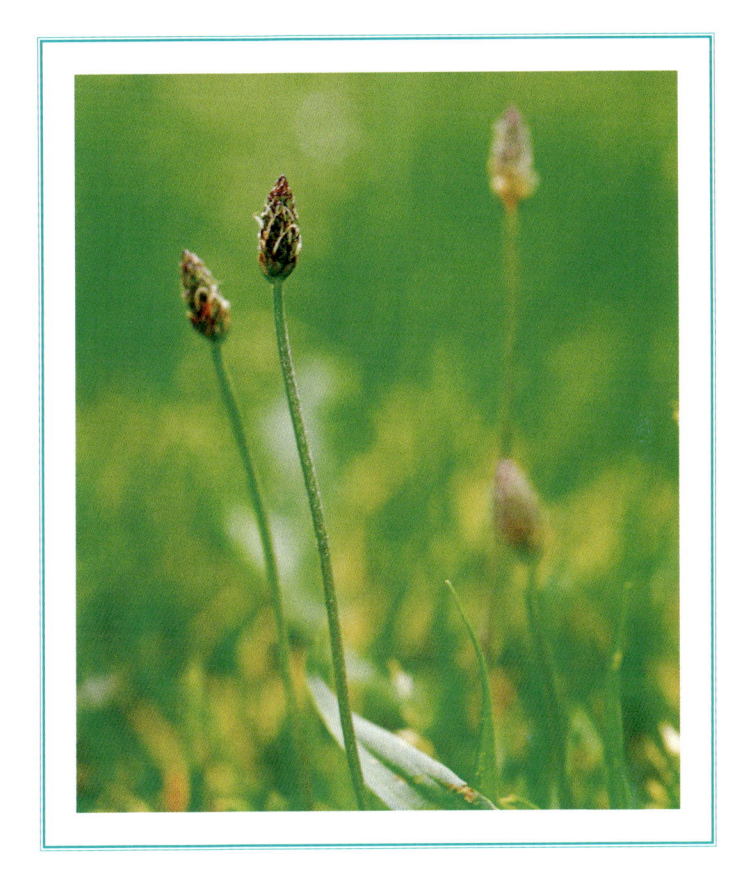

Plantago

33 ASTROLOGICALS

34 ASTROLOGICALS

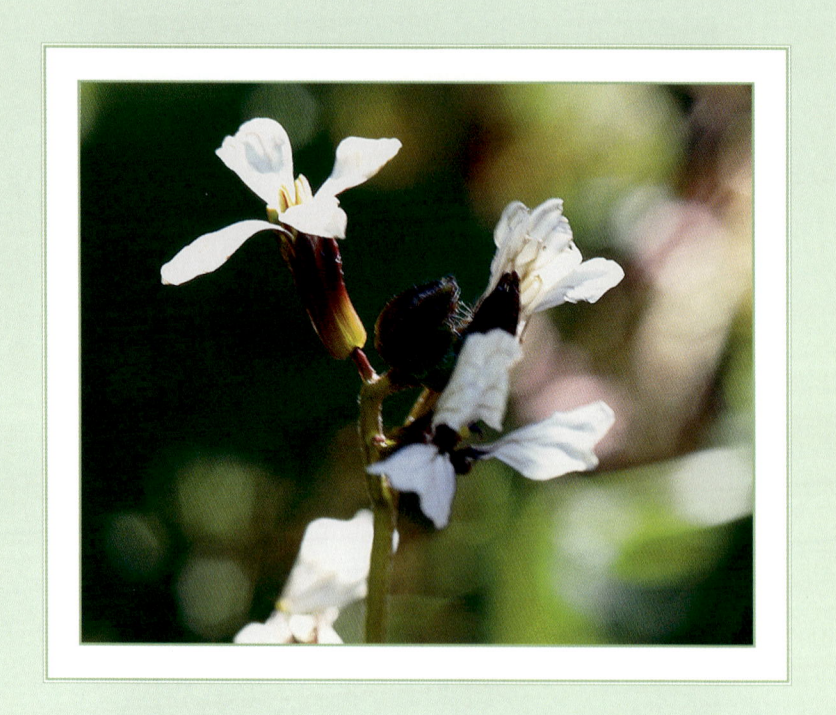

"He who knows what iron is, knows the attributes of Mars. He who knows Mars, knows the qualities of iron."

PARACELSUS (PHILIPPUS VON HOHENHEIM)
16TH CENTURY

Jupiter – PISCES and SAGITTARIUS

JUPITER IS TRADITIONALLY thought of as the planet of good fortune. His feminine sign, Pisces (February 20–March 20), rules the feet and is also associated with excess as a means of escapism, so Pisceans need to guard against addiction, especially with alcohol. The more positive side is that Pisces embodies the benevolent Jupiter characteristics of protectiveness and caring. Jupiter's large appetite for life is also embodied in its masculine sign of Sagittarius (November 23–December 22), the sign of optimism and enthusiasm, but also of excess. This is reflected in Jupiter's rulership of the liver and its function of purifying the blood.

> THE HERBAL CABINET
>
> Red clover was introduced into North America by European settlers, who valued it both as a herbal medicine and as a fodder crop for cattle. It soon became a familiar plant in the hay meadows and roadside verges of New England, and in 1895 it became the official State Flower of Vermont.

Jupiter's herbs are considered to be soothing, cheering, and benevolent. They include red clover (*Trifolium pratense*), which makes an effective poultice for treating athlete's foot, borage, the herbalist's wonder drug, and dandelion, whose roots can be made into an infusion for cleansing the liver.

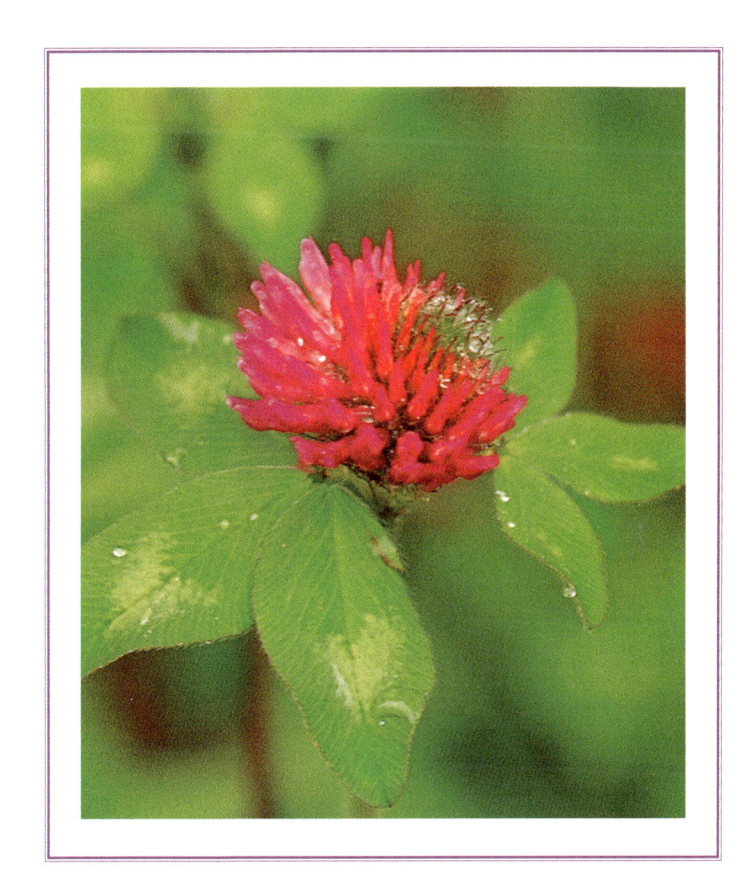

Trifolium pratense

37 ASTROLOGICALS

Dandelion

*B*ecause its jagged leaves were once thought to resemble lion's teeth, this plant became known in France as "dent de lion", and in the sixteenth century this name entered the English language as "dandelion". The dandelion is found throughout the temperate regions of the Northern Hemisphere, and its many useful medicinal effects make it possibly the most widely prescribed plant in Western herbalism.

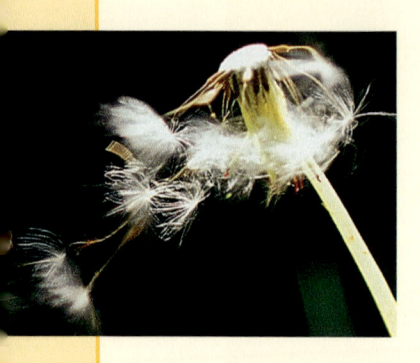

The dandelion is a ground-hugging plant with a cluster of bright green leaves. It produces shiny, purple-tinged stalks that each carry a single bright-yellow flower, and these flowers mature into fuzzy, gossamer-like balls made up of seeds plumed with silky hairs that carry them away in the breeze. It is rich in vitamins and minerals and its leaves are potent diuretics, its roots make an effective liver tonic, and the juice from its stalks can be used to remove warts.

Taraxacum

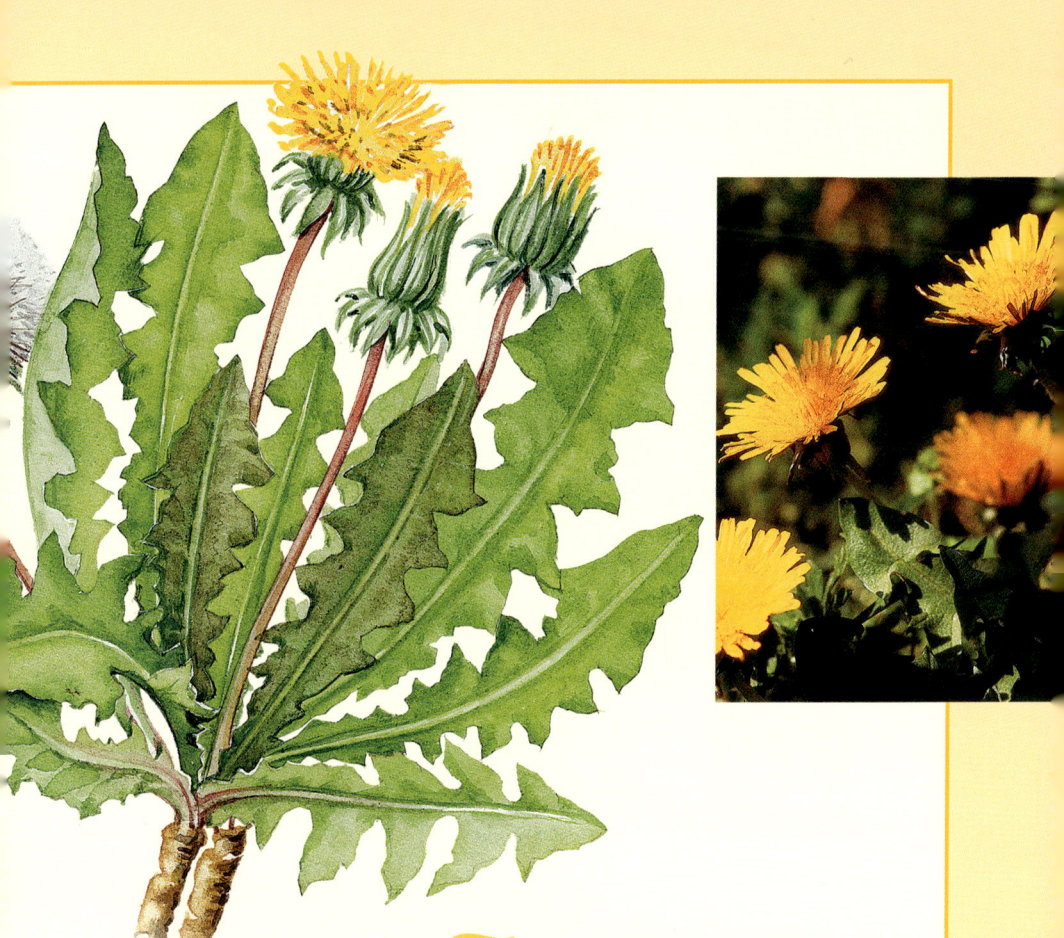

39 ASTROLOGICALS

40 ASTROLOGICALS

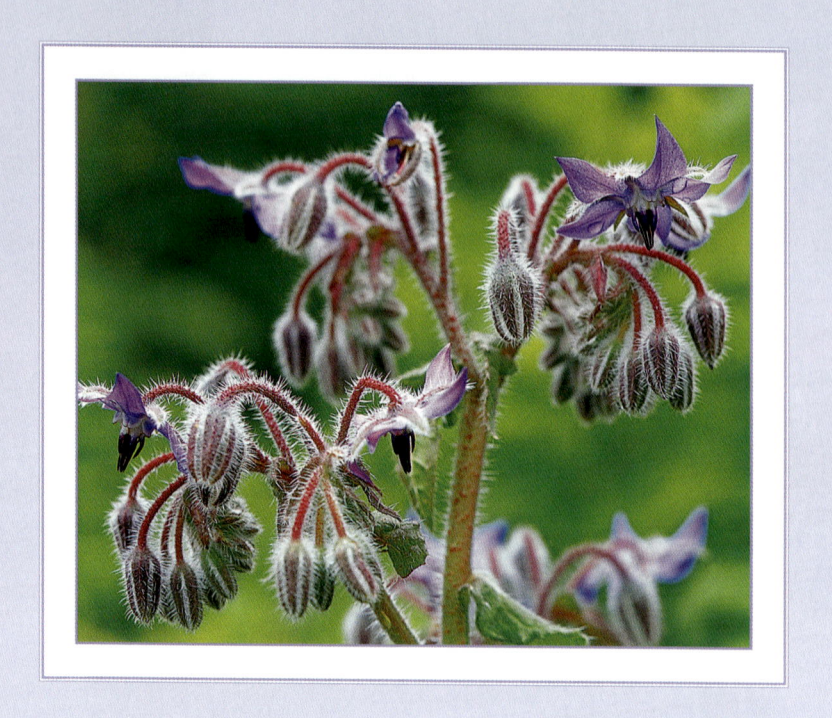

"Jupiter on high laughs at lovers' perjuries,
And orders Aeolus's winds to carry them into
the void."

Ovid
Ars Amatoria
c. 1 BC

Saturn – CAPRICORN and AQUARIUS

TRADITIONALLY, SATURN'S NATURE IS PESSIMISTIC, cold, severe, and controlled, and he rules work, discipline, caution, and thrift. He is also the ruler of all structures and boundaries, including the skeleton and the skin. Saturn's feminine sign, Capricorn (December 23–January 20), embodies many of these key characteristics and Capricorns are known for their endurance, ambition, and sense of purpose. Capricorn rules the bones, especially the knees and teeth, and a poultice made of comfrey (*Symphytum*) can help heal bruised or broken bones.

> **THE HERBAL CABINET**
> The skin- and bone-healing properties of comfrey are largely due to the allantoin it contains. Allantoin is a chemical that softens the skin and encourages cell regeneration, and is a common ingredient of ointments, cosmetic creams, lipsticks, shampoos, toothpastes, and eyedrops.

Saturn's masculine sign is Aquarius (January 21–February 19), which embodies the Saturnian principle of structure and organization, so typical Aquarians are highly disciplined, systematic, cool, and objective. Aquarius rules the legs, especially the ankles, and the circulation so Aquarians often suffer from the cold or circulatory problems, which can be relieved by drinking tea made of shepherd's purse.

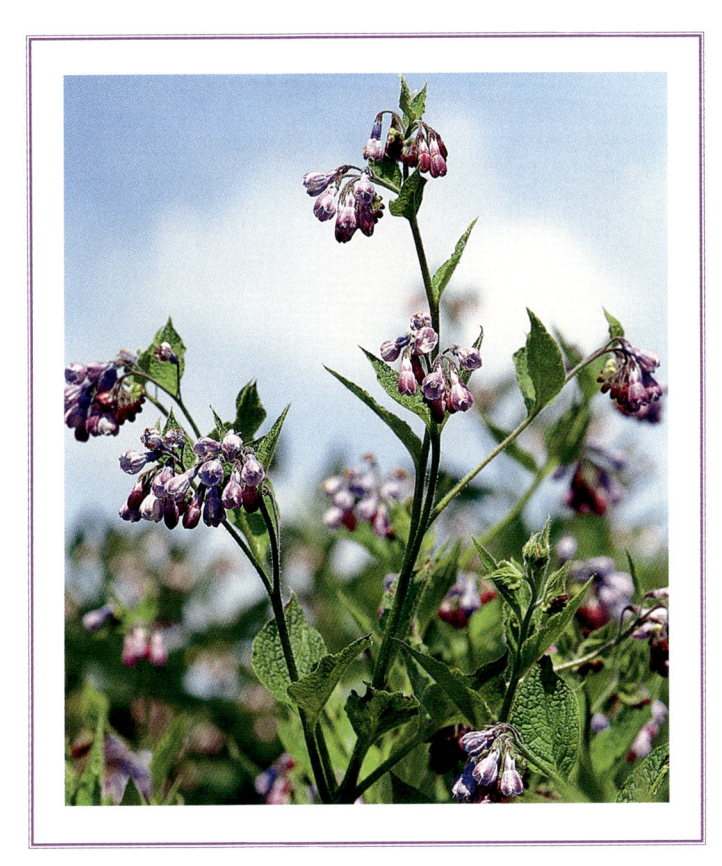

Symphytum

43 ASTROLOGICALS

44 Astrologicals

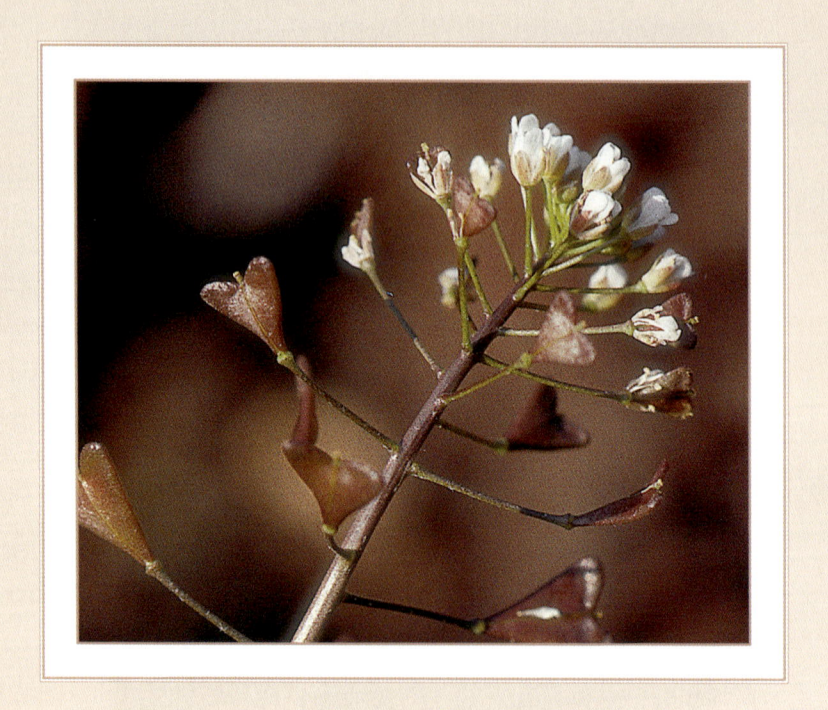

"Let the planet that governs the herb be angular, and the stronger the better; if they can, in herbs of Saturn, let Saturn be in the ascendant."

NICHOLAS CULPEPER
THE ENGLISH PHYSICIAN ENLARGED
1653

Sunflower

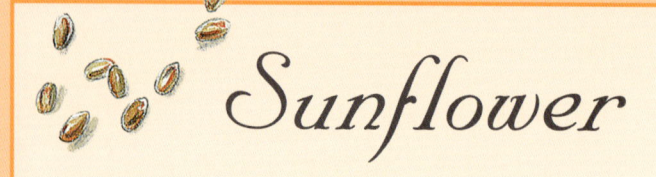

This tall, distinctive plant has large, round, yellow, flower heads, which produce edible seeds that are eaten as snacks and yield a high-quality oil used for cooking, as a salad oil, and for making margarine. The seeds are also used in herbal medicine, to make remedies for bronchial infections, coughs, and colds.

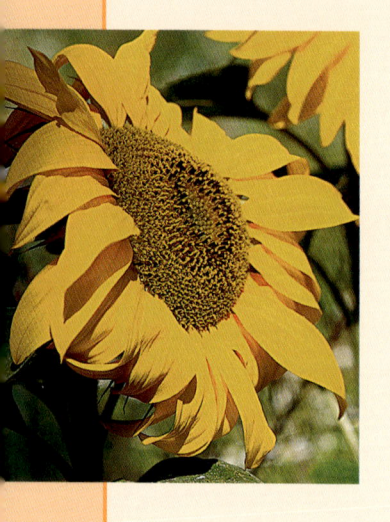

The sunflower was first cultivated in about 3000 BC, by Native Americans. It eventually became a common crop throughout North America, where its seeds were ground to make flour and its oil was used in making bread, and it was brought to Europe by Spanish explorers in the early sixteenth century. Its large-scale cultivation in Europe began in eighteenth-century Russia, where it was very popular because it was not on the Russian Orthodox Church's traditional list of oils and fats that could not be consumed during Lent.

Helianthus

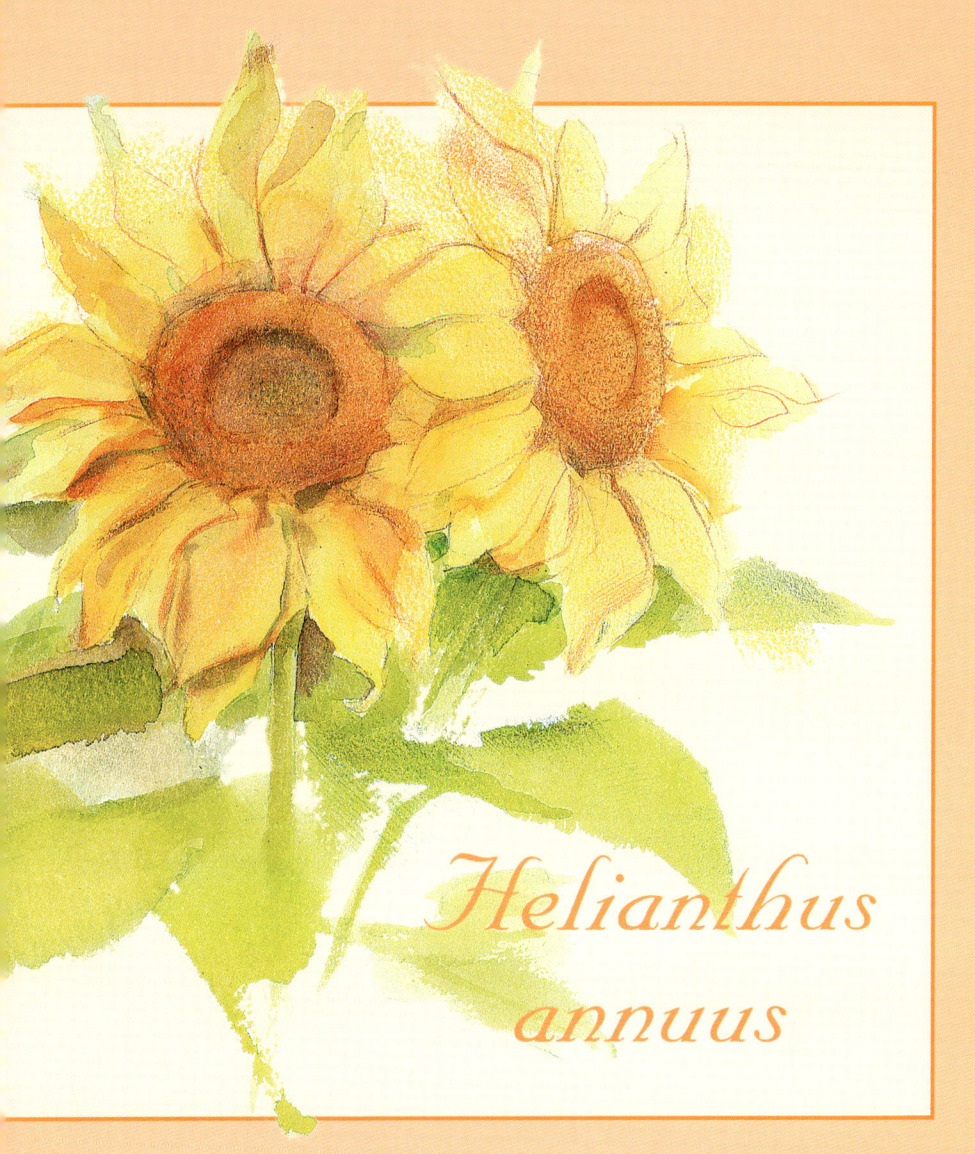

annuus

47 A STROLOGICALS

Making Infusions and Decoctions

THE EASIEST WAY TO PREPARE HERBS for internal use is to make an infusion or a decoction. Infusions, also called teas or tisanes, are the best way of preparing the delicate parts of plants such as the flowers, leaves, and green stems. To make a hot infusion, add 2 tablespoonfuls of dried herbs or 4 tablespoonfuls of fresh herbs to 600 ml (1 pint) of freshly boiled water and leave them to steep for 5 to 10 minutes. For herbs such as marshmallow whose active ingredients are destroyed by heat – use a cold water infusion and soak the herbs for 8 to 12 hours.

> ### THE HERBAL CABINET
> An easy way of preparing herbs for external use is to make a herbal massage oil. Add 10–12 drops of the essential oil of the herb of your choice to 10 teaspoonfuls of a suitable carrier oil, such as sunflower or safflower oil, and mix well. Warm a little oil in your palms and begin your massage.

Use decoctions for preparing the tougher parts of herbs, such as roots, seeds, and barks. First, in a pestle and mortar, break or chop 2 tablespoonfuls of dried herbs or 4 tablespoonfuls of fresh herbs and put them into a pan adding enough cold water to cover. Bring to the boil and simmer for 15 minutes, then strain the mixture and add more water to the liquid to make it up to 600 ml (1 pint).

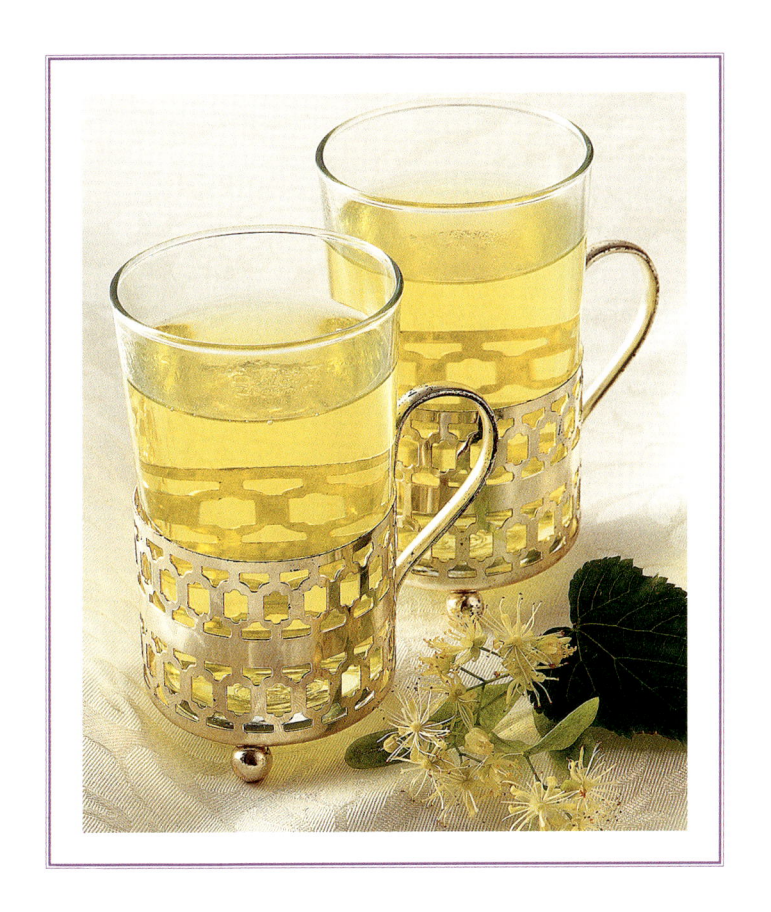

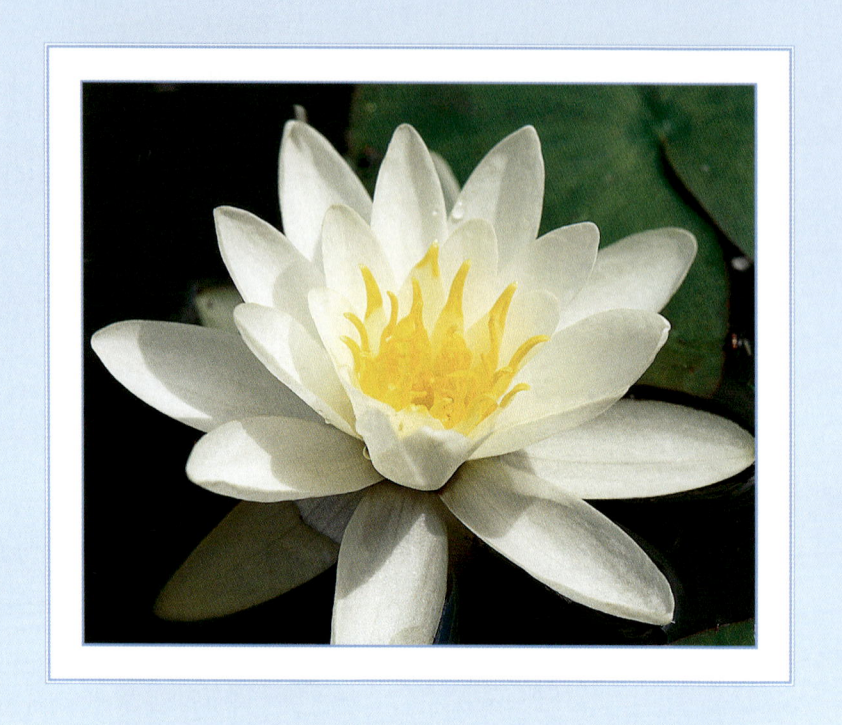

"That orbèd maiden with white fire laden,
    Whom mortals call the Moon,
Glides glimmering o'er my fleece-like floor,
    By the midnight breezes strewn"

PERCY BYSSHE SHELLEY
THE CLOUD
1819

Ginger Tea

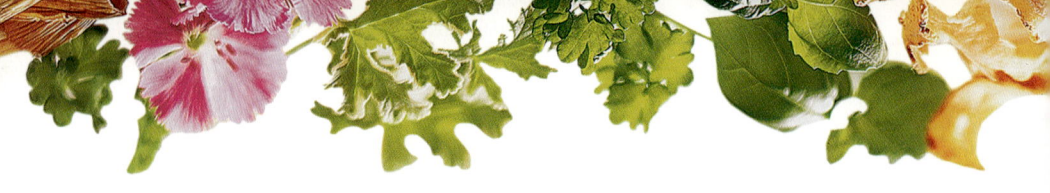

This soothing drink is a lovely remedy for an upset stomach, and for nausea due to travel sickness or morning sickness.

2 thin slices fresh, peeled ginger root
boiling water
1 teasp honey

Put the slices of ginger root into a cup, pour on boiling water, and let it steep for five minutes. Then remove the ginger, stir in a teaspoonful of honey, and sip slowly.

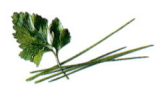

Peppermint Tea

A cup of this refreshing herbal tea will help to relieve indigestion brought on by stress, worry, or simply overeating

1 to 2 teasp dried (or 3 to 4 teasp fresh) peppermint leaves
boiling water

Put the peppermint leaves into a teapot and pour a cupful of boiling water over them. Allow the brew to steep for 10 minutes, then strain it into a cup and sip slowly.

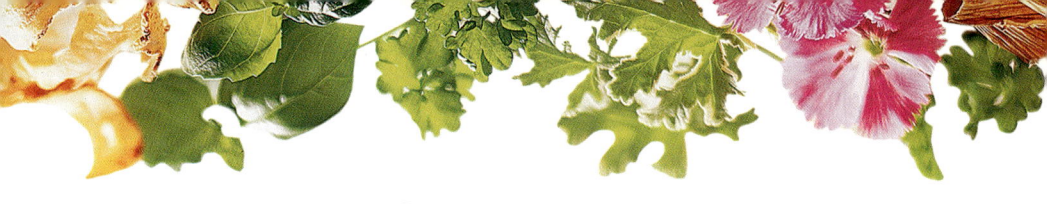

Plantain Tea

Drinking plantain tea three time a day can provide relief from sinusitis, catarrh, and coughs.

**½ teasp dried plantain leaf
boiling water**

To make the tea, soak the plantain leaf in a cupful of boiling water for about 10 minutes, then strain the tea and drink it.

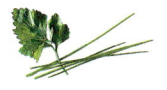

Dandelion Root Tea

A daily cup of dandelion root tea will gently stimulate and cleanse your liver and promote good digestion.

**2 tbsp dried dandelion root
boiling water**

Just simmer the dried dandelion root in a cupful of boiling water for 20 minutes, then strain the liquid into a cup and drink it.

Herb Glossary

BORAGE *(Borago officinalis)*
This popular culinary and medicinal herb originated in the Middle East and was introduced into much of Europe by the Romans. Borage (*below*) is a hardy annual plant that it grows to a height of about 45 cm (18 inches), with thick, hairy stems, wide, fuzzy, grey-green leaves, and bright purple, star-shaped flowers that bloom in May or June.

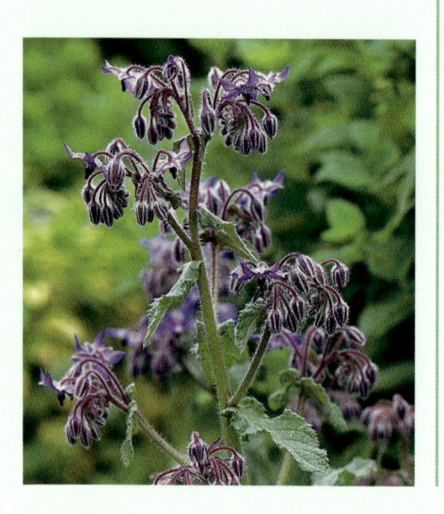

BURDOCK *(Arctium lappa)*
This large, bushy herb has big, coarse leaves that can grow to 30 cm (1 foot) or more in length, and its clusters of purple flowers mature into seed-carrying burrs that cling to clothing and the fur of passing animals. Its leaves and roots are used in herbal medicines and as vegetables and garnishes.

COMFREY *(Symphytum officinale)*
A member of the borage and forget-me-not family, comfrey has a leafy stem 60 to 90 cm (2 to 3 feet) high and drooping clusters of mauve or white flowers. It grows in moist ground throughout Europe and North America, and is valued by herbalists for its ability to heal skin and bone damage. It is also said to help keep skin looking youthful.

DILL *(Anethum graveolens)*
A native of the Mediterranean region and southern Russia, dill (*right*) has a long history as a medicinal herb and an ingredient of magic potions. It grows to

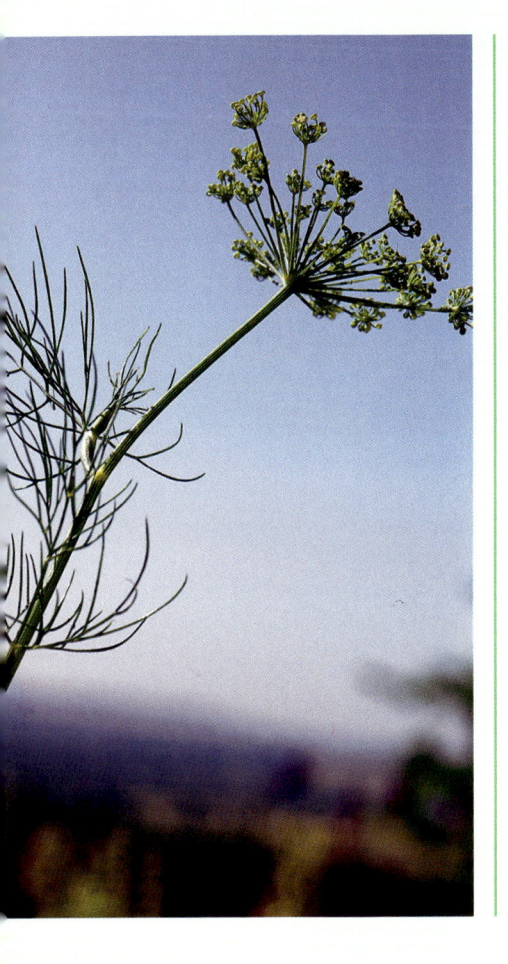

over 60 cm (2 feet) high and produces small, yellow flowers, and its feathery green leaves and tiny seeds are popular culinary flavourings in Scandinavia, Germany, and Central and Eastern Europe.

GINGER *(Zingiber officinalis)*
Prized for its spicy root, ginger is grown commercially in its native southeast Asia and in the southern United States, the West Indies, India, and Africa. Herbalists use ginger root to stimulate the circulation, aid digestion, and relieve nausea, and it is very popular as a flavouring or foodstuff in fresh, dried, powdered, candied, or preserved form.

MARSHMALLOW *(Althaea officinalis)*
The marshmallow has stems that reach a height of 90 to 120 cm (3 or 4 feet), with downy, three- or five-lobed leaves and pale, bluish-pink flowers. It grows in damp meadows, along the banks of tidal rivers, and by the sea. The leaves and flowers are useful for treating coughs and throat infections, while the roots can relieve acid indigestion and diarrhea.

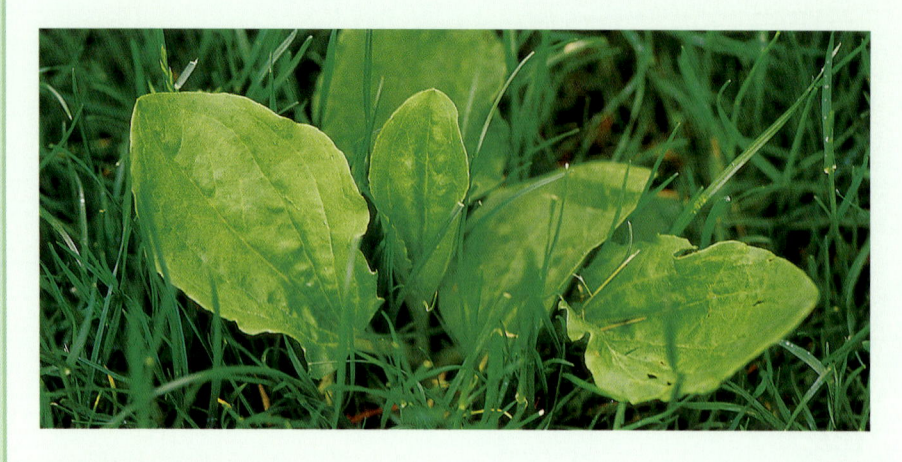

PLANTAIN *(Plantago spp)*
Extremely common plants, plantains (*above*) are found in grassy areas and garden lawns all over Europe. Their leaves lie close to the ground but their stems grow to about 25 cm (10 inches) in height and each one ends in a spike of tiny, grey-brown flowers. The leaves and juice are used to treat sinusitis, catarrh, coughs, and minor bites and wounds.

RED CLOVER *(Trifolium pratense)*
This familiar meadow plant has three-parted, oval leaflets and its reddish-purple flowers have a sweet, vanilla-like scent and are rich in nectar. Red clover is used to treat skin problems including psoriasis, eczema, and athlete's foot, and to relieve coughs, bronchitis, and whooping cough.

ROCKET *(Eruca sativa)*
Closely related to the cabbages and mustards, rocket is an edible herb with a distinctive sharp, peppery flavour. It was once used medicinally as a diuretic and a stimulant, and the ancient Egyptians and Romans regarded it as an aphrodisiac,

but today it is used mainly as a tasty salad herb and to flavour pasta and risotto dishes.

SAFFLOWER *(Carthamus tinctorius)*
The brilliant yellow, orange, or red flowers of the safflower (*right*) are used in herbal medicine to make laxatives and to treat measles, fevers, and skin complaints. Their main use, however, is for making a cheap substitute for saffron (which is the dried stigmas of a crocus, *Crocus sativus*), and their seeds yield an edible oil used in cooking and as a salad oil, and for making margarine.

SHEPHERD'S PURSE *(Capsella bursa-pastoris)*
This common plant grows in temperate regions worldwide, and gets its name from the distinctive shape of its flat seed-pods. It acts as a gentle stimulant for the circulation, but it can also help reduce heavy menstrual bleeding, and in World War I soldiers used its leaves to staunch their wounds.

VALERIAN *(Valeriana officinalis)*
Valerian is widely distributed throughout Europe and northern Asia, where it favours wet or marshy ground and the banks of rivers and ditches. It grows to a height of around 90 cm (3 feet), and its rhizome (the underground part of its stem) and roots are used as a mild sedative and to promote sound sleep.

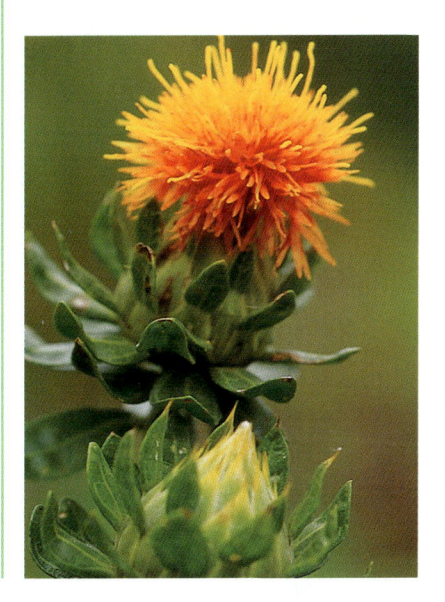

Herbs in Your Garden

HERBS ARE AMONG THE EASIEST OF PLANTS to grow, and herb plants and seeds are readily available. They are relatively untroubled by diseases or insect pests, and you can plant them out in beds, along borders, or the edges of pathways, or in containers or window boxes. All they need is a reasonably sunny location and a light, well-drained soil – if your soil is heavy, fork it well to break it up and mix in some sand, gravel, or compost to lighten its texture.

> ### THE HERBAL CABINET
> It is said that herbs can help to deter pests from neighbouring plants, which is why so many herbs are used in companion planting. For example, garlic, planted next to roses, is said to repel aphids. Try combining your favourite ornamental plants with some aromatic herbs in your garden.

Herbs fall into three main categories – annuals, biennials, and perennials. Annuals have a life cycle of one year, so you will have to grow them again from seed each spring. Biennials last for two years, producing foliage in the first year and flowering in the second, so you will need to sow them again the following year. Some perennials are evergreens, while others die back in winter, but they will all last for several years before you will need to replace them.

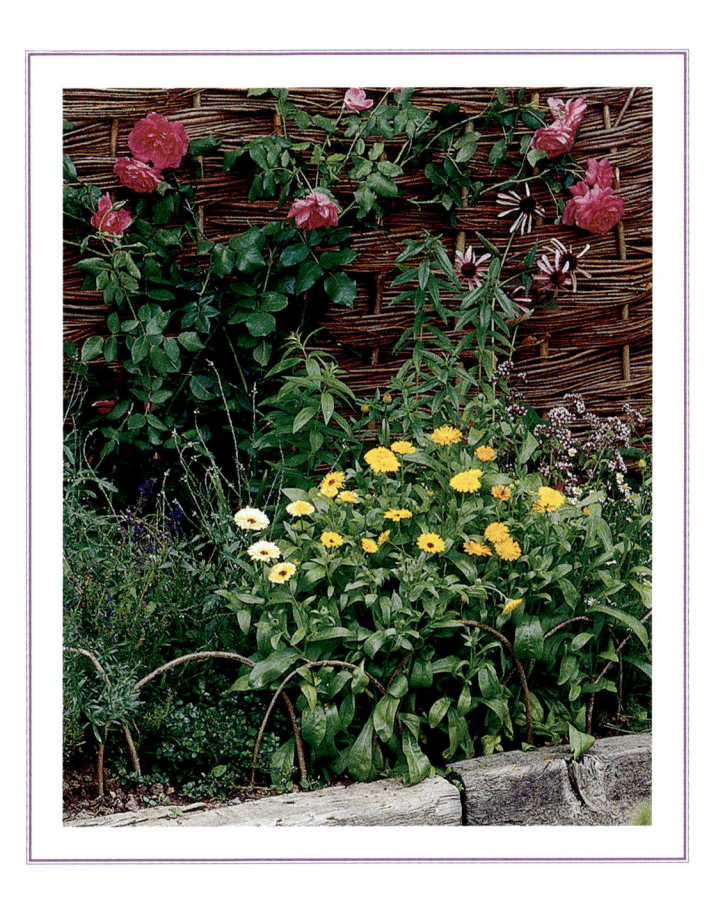

Growing Herbs Indoors

MOST HERBS WILL GROW READILY INDOORS, if they can get enough light and the temperature is reasonably stable at 16 to 21°C (60 to 70°F). Grow them in pots (or a window box) on a sunny windowsill where they will get at least four hours of direct sunlight each day, weather permitting, and turn the pots so that all parts of the plants are exposed to some sunlight on a regular basis.

> **THE HERBAL CABINET**
> Certain herbs thrive indoors, including basil, bay, chives, parsley, rosemary, sage, and thyme. But you don't have to stop at the kitchen door, put some lemon verbena or lavender in your living room or bathroom – every time you brush past, the plant will release its wonderful aroma.

After sunlight, the next most important requirements of indoor herbs are good, well-drained soil and proper watering. Excess moisture is the enemy of herbs' roots, so to ensure proper drainage, use pots with good drainage holes and put a few pieces of broken pot or a layer of gravel at the bottom of each one. Water your herbs regularly, but only when the soil feels dry to the touch; you can add some liquid fertilizer to the water when the plants are growing, but not when they are dormant.

61 ASTROLOGICALS

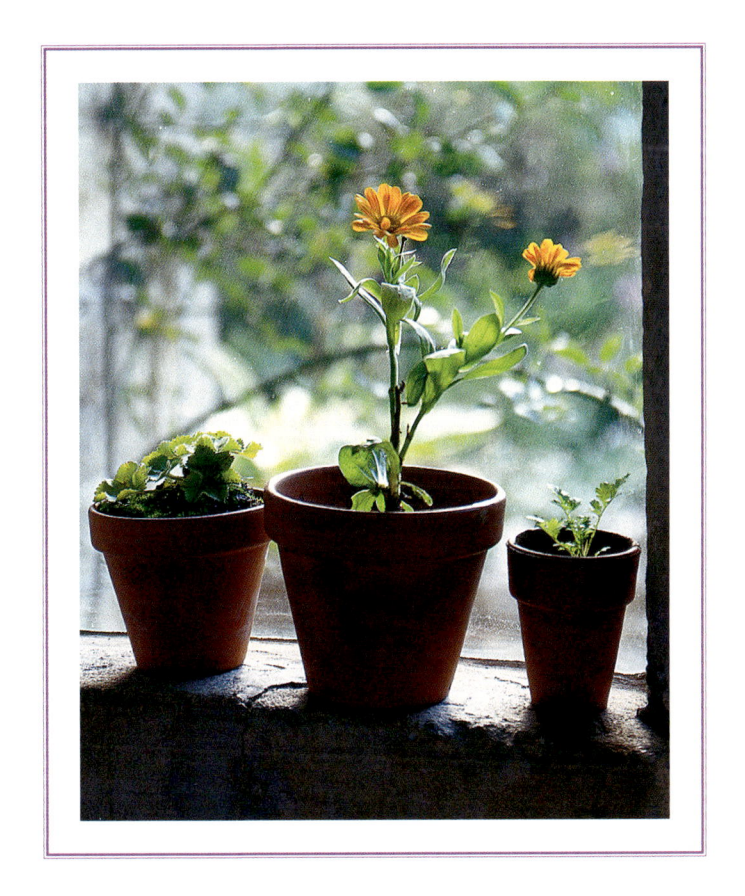

Harvesting Herbs

> **LEGEND & LORE**
>
> *In many ancient cultures women took charge of all matters concerning the planting, growing, and harvesting of food. They sought out plants and roots to eat along with medicinal plants to remedy the ills of their communities. This is because of the deep connection between women and the moon, without which, it was believed, plants and animals could not grow and thrive.*

THE GREAT BENEFIT OF GROWING YOUR OWN HERBS, whether in your garden or indoors, is that they give you an almost constant supply of fresh leaves and sprigs for most of the year. However, there are a few basic rules to observe when it comes to harvesting them.

The best time to pick herb leaves or snip off sprigs is in the morning, after the dew has evaporated (if they are outdoors) but before the Sun has warmed them. Pick only as much as you need for use that day (or for drying or freezing), and avoid any leaves that are discoloured or damaged. Never take more than 10 percent of the total growth from any one plant, and handle the picked herbs gently, because if you crush the leaves or stems the volatile oils that give them their flavour will begin to escape.

63 ASTROLOGICALS

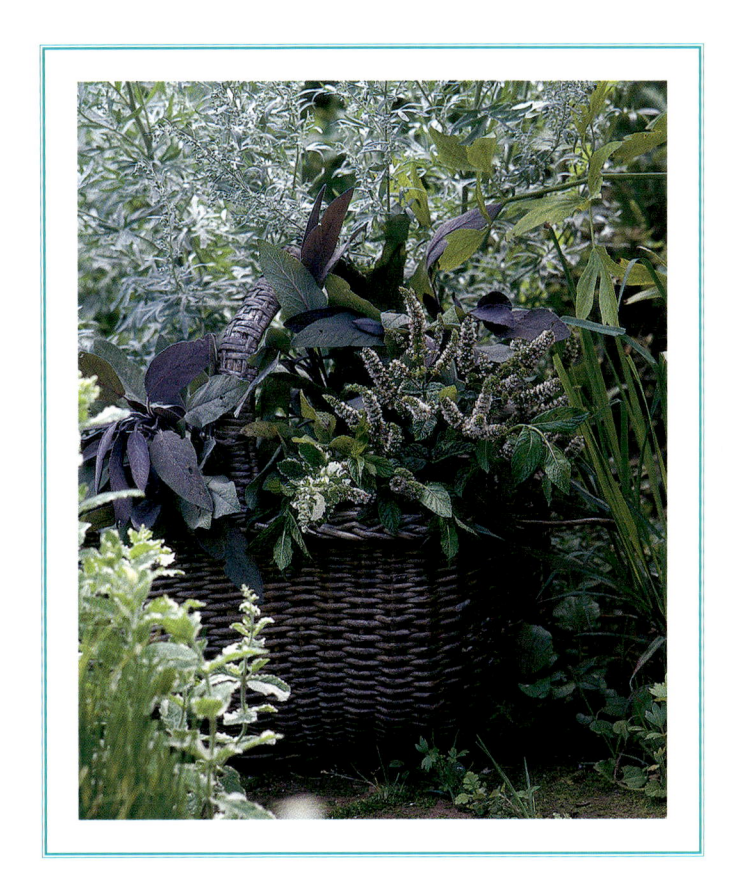

Index

allantoin 42
Aquarius 42
Aries 32
borage 36, 54
burdock 26, 54
calendula (marigold) 10, 29
Cancer 16
Capricorn 42
clover, red 36, 56
comfrey 19, 42, 54
coriander 16
Culpeper, Nicholas 8
dandelion 6, 36, 38–39, 53
decoctions 48
dill 54
Gemini 20
Gerard, John 8
ginger 16, 52, 55
growing herbs 58, 60
harvesting herbs 62
heart trefoil 10
herb safety 6
herbal medicine 6, 8
infusions 48
juniper 10, 12–13, 19

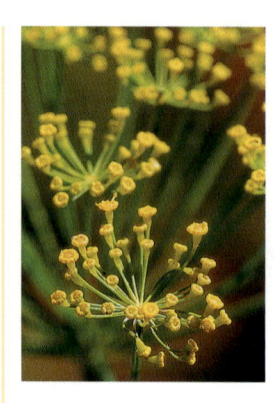

Jupiter 6, 36
Leo 10
Libra 26
Mars 32
marshmallow 26, 29, 48, 55
massage oil 48
Mercury 20
Minthe 22
Moon 16
Parkinson, John 8
peppermint 20, 22–23, 52
Persephone 22

Pisces 36
plantain 32, 53, 56
Pluto 22
Priapus 32
rocket 32, 56
rose 26, 58
rowan 10
safflower 48, 57
Sagittarius 36
Saturn 42
Scorpio 32
shepherd's purse 42, 57
spearmint 22
Sun 6, 10
sunflower 10, 19, 46–47, 48
Taurus 26
teas (tisanes) 48, 52, 53
Thor 13
valerian 20, 57
Venus 26
Virgo 20
water mint 22